ON THE SACRED DISEASE

Hippocrates of Kos
Father of Medicine

Translated: Francis Adams

Edited by: D.P. Curtin

Dalcassian
Publishing
Company

PHILADELPHIA, PA

Library of Congress Cataloging-in-Publication Data

It is thus with regard to the disease called Sacred: it appears to me to be nowise more divine nor more sacred than other diseases, but has a natural cause from the originates like other affections. Men regard its nature and cause as divine from ignorance and wonder, because it is not at all like to other diseases. And this notion of its divinity is kept up by their inability to comprehend it, and the simplicity of the mode by which it is cured, for men are freed from it by purifications and incantations. But if it is reckoned divine because it is wonderful, instead of one there are many diseases which would be sacred; for, as I will show, there are others no less wonderful and prodigious, which nobody imagines to be sacred. The quotidian, tertian, and quartan fevers, seem to me no less sacred and divine in their origin than this disease, although they are not reckoned so wonderful. And I see men become mad and demented from no manifest cause, and at the same time doing many things out of place; and I have known many persons in sleep groaning and crying out, some in a state of suffocation, some jumping up and fleeing out of doors, and deprived of their reason until they awaken, and afterward becoming well and rational as before, although they be pale and weak; and this will happen not once but frequently. And there are many and various things of the like kind, which it would be tedious to state particularly.

They who first referred this malady to the gods appear to me to have been just such persons as the conjurors, purificators, mountebanks, and charlatans now are, who give themselves out for being excessively religious, and as knowing more than other people. Such persons, then, using the divinity as a pretext and screen of their own inability to of their own inability to afford any assistance, have given out that the disease is sacred, adding suitable reasons for this opinion, they have instituted a mode of treatment which is safe for themselves, namely, by applying purifications and incantations, and enforcing abstinence from baths and many articles of food which are unwholesome to men in diseases. Of sea substances, the surmullet, the blacktail, the mullet, and the eel; for these are the fishes most to be guarded against. And of fleshes, those of the goat, the stag, the sow, and the dog: for these are the kinds of flesh which are aptest to disorder the bowels. Of fowls, the cock, the turtle, and the bustard, and such others as are reckoned to be particularly strong. And of potherbs, mint, garlic, and onions; for what is acrid does not agree with a weak person. And they forbid to have a black robe, because black is expressive of death; and to sleep on a goat's skin, or to wear it, and to put one foot upon another, or one hand upon another; for all these things are held to be hindrances to the cure. All these they enjoin with reference to its divinity, as if possessed of more knowledge, and announcing beforehand other causes so that if the person should recover, theirs would be the honor and credit; and if he should die, they would have a certain defense, as if the gods, and not they, were to blame, seeing they had administered nothing either to eat or drink as medicines, nor had overheated him with baths, so as to prove the cause of what had happened. But I am of opinion that (if this were true) none of the Libyans, who live in the interior, would be free from this disease, since they all sleep on goats' skins, and live upon goats' flesh; neither have they couch, robe, nor shoe that is not made of goat's skin, for they have no other herds but goats and oxen. But if these things, when administered in food, aggravate the disease, and if it be cured by abstinence from them, godhead is not the cause at all; nor will purifications be of any avail, but it is the food which is beneficial and prejudicial, and the influence of the divinity vanishes.

Thus, they who try to cure these maladies in this way, appear to me neither to reckon them sacred nor divine. For when they are removed by such purifications, and this method of cure, what is to prevent them from being brought upon men and induced by other devices similar to these? So that the cause is no longer divine, but human. For whoever is able, by purifications conjurations, to drive away such an affection, will be able, by other practices, to excite it; and, according to this view, its divine nature is entirely done away with. By such sayings and doings, they profess to be possessed of superior knowledge, and deceive mankind by enjoining lustrations and purifications upon them, while their discourse turns upon the divinity and the godhead. And yet it would appear to me that their discourse savors not of piety, as they suppose, but rather of impiety, and as if there were no gods, and that what they hold to be holy and divine, were impious and unholy. This I will now explain.

For, if they profess to know how to bring down the moon, darken the sun, induce storms and fine weather, and rains and droughts, and make the sea and land unproductive, and so forth, whether they arrogate this power as being derived from mysteries or any other knowledge or consideration, they appear to me to practice impiety, and either to fancy that there are no gods, or, if there are, that they have no ability to ward off any of the greatest evils. How, then, are they not enemies to the gods? For if a man by magical arts and sacrifices will bring down the moon, and darken the sun, and induce storms, or fine weather, I should not believe that there was anything divine, but human, in these things, provided the power of the divine were overpowered by human knowledge and subjected to it. But perhaps it will be said, these things are not so, but, not withstanding, men being in want of the means of life, invent many and various things, and devise many contrivances for all other things, and for this disease, in every phase of the disease, assigning the cause to a god. Nor do they remember the same things once, but frequently. For, if they imitate a goat, or grind their teeth, or if their right side be convulsed, they say that the mother of the gods is the cause. But if they speak in a sharper and more intense tone, they resemble this state to a horse, and say that Poseidon is the cause. Or if any excrement be passed, which is often the case, owing to the violence of the disease, the appellation of Enodia is adhibited; or, if it be passed in smaller and denser masses, like bird's, it is said to be from Apollo Nomius. But if foam be emitted by the mouth, and the patient kick with his feet, Ares then gets the blame. But terrors which happen during the night, and fevers, and delirium, and jumpings out of bed, and frightful apparitions, and fleeing away,-all these they hold to be the plots of Hecate, and the invasions the and use purifications and incantations, and, as appears to me, make the divinity to be most wicked and most impious. For they purify those laboring under this disease, with the same sorts of blood and the other means that are used in the case of those who are stained with crimes, and of malefactors, or who have been enchanted by men, or who have done any wicked act; who ought to do the very reverse, namely, sacrifice and pray, and, bringing gifts to the temples, supplicate the gods. But now they do none of these things, but purify; and some of the purifications they conceal in the earth, and some they throw into the sea, and some they carry to the mountains where no one can touch or tread upon them. But these they ought to take to the temples and present to the god, if a god be the cause of the disease. Neither truly do I count it a worthy opinion to hold that the body of man is polluted by god, the most impure by the most holy; for were it defiled, or did it suffer from any other thing, it would be like to be purified and sanctified rather than polluted by god. For it is the divinity which purifies and sanctifies the greatest of offenses and the most wicked, and which proves our protection from them. And we mark out the boundaries of the temples and the groves of the gods, so that no one may pass them unless he be pure, and when we enter them we are sprinkled with holy water, not as being polluted, but as laying aside any other pollution which we formerly had. And thus it appears to me to hold, with regard to purifications.

But this disease seems to me to be no more divine than others; but it has its nature such as other diseases have, and a cause whence it originates, and its nature and cause are divine only just as much as all others are, and it is curable no less than the others, unless when, the from of time, it is confirmed, and has became stronger than the remedies applied. Its origin is hereditary, like that of other diseases. For if a phlegmatic person be born of a phlegmatic, and a bilious of a bilious, and a phthisical of a phthisical, and one having spleen disease, of another having disease of the spleen, what is to hinder it from happening that where the father and mother were subject to this disease, certain of their offspring should be so affected also? As the semen comes from all parts of the body, healthy particles will come from healthy parts, and unhealthy from unhealthy parts. And another great proof that it is in nothing more divine than other diseases is, that it occurs in those who are of a phlegmatic constitution, but does not attack the bilious. Yet, if it were more divine than the others, this disease ought to befall all alike, and make no distinction between the bilious and phlegmatic.

But the brain is the cause of this affection, as it is of other very great diseases, and in what manner and from what cause it is formed, I will now plainly declare. The brain of man, as in all other animals, is double, and a thin membrane divides it through the middle, and therefore the pain is not always in the same part of the head; for sometimes it is situated on either side, and sometimes the whole is affected; and veins run toward it from all parts of the body, many of which are small, but two are thick, the one from the liver, and the other from the spleen. And it is thus with regard to the one from the liver: a portion of it runs downward through the parts on the side, near the kidneys and the psoas muscles, to the inner part of the thigh, and extends to the foot. It is called vena cava. The other runs upward by the right veins and the lungs, and divides into branches for the heart and the right arm. The remaining part of it rises upward across the clavicle to the right side of the neck, and is superficial so as to be seen; near the ear it is concealed, and there it divides; its thickest, largest, and most hollow part ends in the brain; another small vein goes to the right ear, another to the right eye, and another to the nostril. Such are the distributions of the hepatic vein. And a vein from the spleen is distributed on the left side, upward and downward, like that from the liver, but more slender and feeble.

By these veins we draw in much breath, since they are the spiracles of our bodies inhaling air to themselves and distributing it to the rest of the body, and to the smaller veins, and they and afterwards exhale it. For the breath cannot be stationary, but it passes upward and downward, for if stopped and intercepted, the part where it is stopped becomes powerless. In proof of this, when, in sitting or lying, the small veins are compressed, so that the breath from the larger vein does not pass into them, the part is immediately seized with numbness; and it is so likewise with regard to the other veins.

This malady, then, affects phlegmatic people, but not bilious. It begins to be formed while the foetus is still in utero. For the brain, like the other organs, is depurated and grows before birth. If, then, in this purgation it be properly and moderately depurated, and neither more nor less than what is proper be secreted from it, the head is thus in the most healthy condition. If the secretion (melting) the from the brain be greater than natural, the person, when he grows up, will have his head diseased, and full of noises, and will neither be able to endure the sun nor cold. Or, if the melting take place from any one part, either from the eye or ear, or if a vein has become slender, that part will be deranged in proportion to the melting. Or, should depuration not take place, but congestion accumulate in the brain, it necessarily becomes phlegmatic. And such children as have an eruption of ulcers on the head, on the ears, and along the rest of the body, with copious discharges of saliva and mucus,-these, in after life, enjoy best health; for in this way the phlegm which ought to have been purged off in the womb, is discharged and cleared away, and persons so purged, for the most part, are not subject to attacks of this disease. But such as have had their skin free from eruptions, and have had no discharge of saliva or mucus, nor have undergone the proper purgation in the womb, these persons run the risk of being seized with this disease.

But should the defluxion make its way to the heart, the person is seized with palpitation and asthma, the chest becomes diseased, and some also have curvature of the spine. For when a defluxion of cold phlegm takes place on the lungs and heart, the blood is chilled, and the veins, being violently chilled, palpitate in the lungs and heart, and the heart palpitates, so that from this necessity asthma and orthopnoea supervene. For it does not receive the spirits as much breath as he needs until the defluxion of phlegm be mastered, and being heated is distributed to the veins, then it ceases from its palpitation and difficulty of breathing, and this takes place as soon as it obtains an abundant supply; and this will be more slowly, provided the defluxion be more abundant, or if it be less, more quickly. And if the defluxions be more condensed, the epileptic attacks will be more frequent, but otherwise if it be rarer. Such are the symptoms when the defluxion is upon the lungs and heart; but if it be upon the bowels, the person is attacked with diarrhoea.

And if, being shut out from all these outlets, its defluxion be determined to the veins I have formerly mentioned, the patient loses his speech, and chokes, and foam issues by the mouth, the teeth are fixed, the hands are contracted, the eyes distorted, he becomes insensible, and in some cases the bowels are evacuated. And these symptoms occur sometimes on the left side, sometimes on the right, and sometimes in both. The cause of everyone of these symptoms I will now explain. The man becomes speechless when the phlegm, suddenly descending into the veins, shuts out the air, and does not admit it either to the brain or to the vena cava, or to the ventricles, but interrupts the inspiration. For when a person draws in air by the mouth and nostrils, the breath goes first to the brain, then the greater part of it to the internal cavity, and part to the lungs, and part to the veins, and from them it is distributed to the other parts of the body along the veins; and whatever passes to the stomach cools, and does nothing more; and so also with regard to the lungs. But the air which enters the veins is of use (to the body) by entering the brain and its ventricles, and thus it imparts sensibility and motion to all the members, so that when the veins are excluded from the air by the phlegm and do not receive it, the man loses his speech and intellect, and the hands become powerless, and are contracted, the blood stopping and not being diffused, as it was wont; and the eyes are distorted owing to the veins being excluded from the air; and they palpitate; and froth from the lungs issues by the mouth. For when the breath does not find entrance to him, he foams and sputters like a dying person. And the bowels are evacuated in consequence of the violent suffocation; and the suffocation is produced when the liver and stomach ascend to the diaphragm, and the mouth of the stomach is shut up; this takes place when the breath does not enter by the mouth, as it is wont. The patient kicks with his feet when the air is shut up in the lungs and cannot find an outlet, owing to the phlegm; and rushing by the blood upward and downward, it occasions convulsions and pain, and therefore he kicks with his feet. All these symptoms he endures when the cold phlegm passes into the warm blood, for it congeals and stops the blood. And if the deflexion be copious and thick, it immediately proves fatal to him, for by its cold it prevails over the blood and congeals it; or, if it be less, it in the first place obtains the mastery, and stops the respiration; and then in the course of time, when it is diffused along the veins and mixed with much warm blood, it is thus overpowered, the veins receive the air, and the patient recovers his senses.

Of little children who are seized with this disease, the greater part die, provided the defluxion be copious and humid, for the veins being slender cannot admit the phlegm, owing to its thickness and abundance; but the blood is cooled and congealed, and the child immediately dies. But if the phlegm be in small quantity, and make a defluxion into both the veins, or to those on either side, the children survive, but exhibit notable marks of the disorder; for either the mouth is drawn aside, or an eye, the neck, or a hand, wherever a vein being filled with phlegm loses its tone, and is attenuated, and the part of the body connected with this vein is necessarily rendered weaker and defective. But for the most it affords relief for a longer interval; for the child is no longer seized with these attacks, if once it has contracted this impress of the disease, in consequence of which the other veins are necessarily affected, and to a certain degree attenuated, so as just to admit the air, but no longer to permit the influx of phlegm. However, the parts are proportionally enfeebled whenever the veins are in an unhealthy state. When in striplings the defluxion is small and to the right side, they recover without leaving any marks of the disease, but there is danger of its becoming habitual, and even increasing if not treated by suitable remedies. Thus, or very nearly so, is the case when it attacks children.

To persons of a more advanced age, it neither proves fatal, nor produces distortions. For their veins are capacious and are filled with hot blood; and therefore the phlegm can neither prevail nor cool the blood, so as to coagulate it, but it is quickly overpowered and mixed with the blood, and thus the veins receive the air, and sensibility remains; and, owing to their strength, the aforesaid symptoms are less likely to seize them. But when this disease attacks very old people, it therefore proves fatal, or induces paraplegia, because the veins are empty, and the blood scanty, thin, and watery. When, therefore, the defluxion is copious, and the season winter, it proves fatal; for it chokes up the exhalents, and coagulates the blood if the defluxion be to both sides; but if to either, it merely induces paraplegia. For the blood being thin, cold, and scanty, cannot prevail over the but being itself overpowered, it is coagulated, so that those parts in which the blood is corrupted, lose their strength.

The flux is to the right rather than to the left because the veins there are more capacious and numerous than on the left side, for on the one side they spring from the liver, and on the other from the spleen. The defluxion and melting down take place most especially in the case of children in whom the head is heated either by the sun or by fire, or if the brain suddenly contract a rigor, and then the phlegm is excreted. For it is melted down by the heat and diffusion of the but it is excreted by the congealing and contracting of it, and thus a defluxion takes place. And in some this is the cause of the disease, and in others, when the south wind quickly succeeds to northern breezes, it suddenly unbinds and relaxes the brain, which is contracted and weak, so that there is an inundation of phlegm, and thus the defluxion takes place. The defluxion also takes place in consequence of fear, from any hidden cause, if we are the at any person's calling aloud, or while crying, when one cannot quickly recover one's breath, such as often happens to children. When any of these things occur, the body immediately shivers, the person becoming speechless cannot draw his breath, but the breath (pneuma) stops, the brain is contracted, the blood stands still, and thus the excretion and defluxion of the phlegm take place. In children, these are the causes of the attack at first. But to old persons winter is most inimical. For when the head and brain have been heated at a great fire, and then the person is brought into cold and has a rigor, or when from cold he comes into warmth, and sits at the fire, he is apt to suffer in the same way, and thus he is seized in the manner described above. And there is much danger of the same thing occurring, if his head be exposed to the sun, but less so in summer, as the changes are not sudden. When a person has passed the twentieth year of his life, this disease is not apt to seize him, unless it has become habitual from childhood, or at least this is rarely or never the case. For the veins are filled with blood, and the brain consistent and firm, so that it does not run down into the veins, or if it do, it does not master the blood, which is copious and hot.

But when it has gained strength from one's childhood, and become habitual, such a person usually suffers attacks, and is seized with them in changes of the winds, especially in south winds, and it is difficult of removal. For the brain becomes more humid than natural, and is inundated with phlegm, so that the defluxions become more frequent, and the phlegm can no longer be the nor the brain be dried up, but it becomes wet and humid. This you may ascertain in particular, from beasts of the flock which are seized with this disease, and more especially goats, for they are most frequently attacked with it. If you will cut open the head, you will find the brain humid, full of sweat, and having a bad smell. And in this way truly you may see that it is not a god that injures the body, but disease. And so it is with man. For when the disease has prevailed for a length of time, it is no longer curable, as the brain is corroded by the phlegm, and melted, and what is melted down becomes water, and surrounds the brain externally, and overflows it; wherefore they are more frequently and readily seized with the disease. And therefore the disease is protracted, because the influx is thin, owing to its quantity, and is immediately overpowered by the blood and heated all through.

But such persons as are habituated to the disease know beforehand when they are about to be seized and flee from men; if their own house be at hand, they run home, but if not, to a deserted place, where as few persons as possible will see them falling, and they immediately cover themselves up. This they do from shame of the affection, and not from fear of the divinity, as many suppose. And little children at first fall down wherever they may happen to be, from inexperience. But when they have been often seized, and feel its approach beforehand, they flee to their mothers, or to any other person they are acquainted with, from terror and dread of the affection, for being still infants they do not know yet what it is to be ashamed.

Therefore, they are attacked during changes of the winds, and especially south winds, then also with north winds, and afterwards also with the others. These are the strongest winds, and the most opposed to one another, both as to direction and power. For, the north wind condenses the air, and separates from it whatever is muddy and nebulous, and renders it clearer and brighter, and so in like manner also, all the winds which arise from the sea and other waters; for they extract the humidity and nebulosity from all objects, and from men themselves, and therefore it (the north wind) is the most wholesome of the winds. But the effects of the south are the very reverse. For in the first place it begins by melting and diffusing the condensed air, and therefore it does not blow strong at first, but is gentle at the commencement, because it is not able at once to overcome the and compacted air, which yet in a while it dissolves. It produces the same effects upon the land, the sea, the fountains, the wells, and on every production which contains humidity, and this, there is in all things, some more, some less. For all these feel the effects of this wind, and from clear they become cloudy, from cold, hot; from dry, moist; and whatever ear then vessels are placed upon the ground, filled with wine or any other fluid, are affected with the south wind, and undergo a change. And the a change. And the sun, and the moon, it renders blunter appearance than they naturally are. When, then, it possesses such powers over things so great and strong, and the body is made to feel and undergo changes in the changes of the winds, it necessarily follows that the brain should be disolved and overpowered with moisture, and that the veins should become more relaxed by the south winds, and that by the north the healthiest portion of the brain should become contracted, while the most morbid and humid is secreted, and overflows externally, and that catarrhs should thus take place in the changes of these winds. Thus is this disease formed and prevails from those things which enter into and go out of the body, and it is not more difficult to understand or to cure than the others, neither is it more divine than other diseases.

Men ought to know that from nothing else but the brain come joys, delights, laughter and sports, and sorrows, griefs, despondency, and lamentations. And by this, in an especial manner, we acquire wisdom and knowledge, and see and hear, and know what are foul and what are fair, what are bad and what are good, what are sweet, and what unsavory; some we discriminate by habit, and some we perceive by their utility. By this we distinguish objects of relish and disrelish, according to the seasons; and the same things do not always please us. And by the same organ we become mad and delirious, and fears and terrors assail us, some by night, and some by day, and dreams and untimely wanderings, and cares that are not suitable, and ignorance of present circumstances, desuetude, and unskilfulness. All these things we endure from the brain, when it is not healthy, but is more hot, more cold, more moist, or more dry than natural, or when it suffers any other preternatural and unusual affection. And we become mad from its humidity. For when it is more moist than natural, it is necessarily put into motion, and the affection being moved, neither the sight nor hearing can be at rest, and the tongue speaks in accordance with the sight and hearing.

As long as the brain is at rest, the man enjoys his reason, but the depravement of the brain arises from phlegm and bile, either of which you may recognize in this manner: Those who are mad from phlegm are quiet, and do not cry out nor make a noise; but those from bile are vociferous, malignant, and will not be quiet, but are always doing something improper. If the madness be constant, these are the causes thereof. But if terrors and fears assail, they are connected with derangement of the brain, and derangement is owing to its being heated. And it is heated by bile when it is determined to the brain along the bloodvessels running from the trunk; and fear is present until it returns again to the veins and trunk, when it ceases. He is grieved and troubled when the brain is unseasonably cooled and contracted beyond its wont. This it suffers from phlegm, and from the same affection the patient becomes oblivious. He calls out and screams at night when the brain is suddenly heated. The bilious endure this. But the phlegmatic are not heated, except when much blood goes to the brain, and creates an ebullition. Much blood passes along the aforesaid veins. But when the man happens to see a frightful dream and is in fear as if awake, then his face is in a greater glow, and the eyes are red when the patient is in fear. And the understanding meditates doing some mischief, and thus it is affected in sleep. But if, when awakened, he returns to himself, and the blood is again distributed along the veins, it ceases.

In these ways I am of the opinion that the brain exercises the greatest power in the man. This is the interpreter to us of those things which emanate from the air, when the brain happens to be in a sound state.

But the air supplies sense to it. And the eyes, the ears, the tongue and the feet, administer such things as the brain cogitates. For in as much as it is supplied with air, does it impart sense to the body. It is the brain which is the messenger to the understanding. For when the man draws the breath into himself, it passes first to the brain, and thus the air is distributed to the rest of the body, leaving in the brain its acme, and whatever has sense and understanding. For if it passed first to the body and last to the brain, then having left in the flesh and veins the judgment, when it reached the brain it would be hot, and not at all pure, but mixed with the humidity from flesh and blood, so as to be no longer pure.

Wherefore, I say, that it is the brain which interprets the understanding. But the diaphragm has obtained its name (frenes) from accident and usage, and not from reality or nature, for I know no power which it possesses, either as to sense or understanding, except that when the man is affected with unexpected joy or sorrow, it throbs and produces palpitations, owing to its thinness, and as having no belly to receive anything good or bad that may present themselves to it, but it is thrown into commotion by both these, from its natural weakness. It then perceives beforehand none of those things which occur in the body, but has received its name vaguely and without any proper reason, like the parts about the heart, which are called auricles, but which contribute nothing towards hearing. Some say that we think with the heart, and that this is the part which is grieved, and experiences care. But it is not so; only it contracts like the diaphragm, and still more so for the same causes. For veins from all parts of the body run to it, and it has valves, so as to as to perceive if any pain or pleasurable emotion befall the man. For when grieved the body necessarily shudders, and is contracted, and from excessive joy it is affected in like manner. Wherefore the heart and the diaphragm are particularly sensitive, they have nothing to do, however, with the operations of the understanding, but of all but of all these the brain is the cause. Since, then, the brain, as being the primary seat of sense and of the spirits, perceives whatever occurs in the body, if any change more powerful than usual take place in the air, owing to the seasons, the brain becomes changed by the state of the air. For, on this account, the brain first perceives, because, I say, all the most acute, most powerful, and most deadly diseases, and those which are most difficult to be understood by the inexperienced, fall upon the brain.

And the disease called the Sacred arises from causes as the others, namely, those things which enter and quit the body, such as cold, the sun, and the winds, which are ever changing and are never at rest. And these things are divine, so that there is no necessity for making a distinction, and holding this disease to be more divine than the others, but all are divine, and all human. And each has its own peculiar nature and power, and none is of an ambiguous nature, or irremediable. And the most of them are curable by the same means as those by which any other thing is food to one, and injurious to another. Thus, then, the physician should understand and distinguish the season of each, so that at one time he may attend to the nourishment and increase, and at another to abstraction and diminution. And in this disease as in all others, he must strive not to feed the disease, but endeavor to wear it out by administering whatever is most opposed to each disease, and not that which favors and is allied to it. For by that which is allied to it, it gains vigor and increase, but it wears out and disappears under the use of that which is opposed to it. But whoever is acquainted with such a change in men, and can render a man humid and dry, hot and cold by regimen, could also cure this disease, if he recognizes the proper season for administering his remedies, without minding purifications, spells, and all other illiberal practices of a like kind.

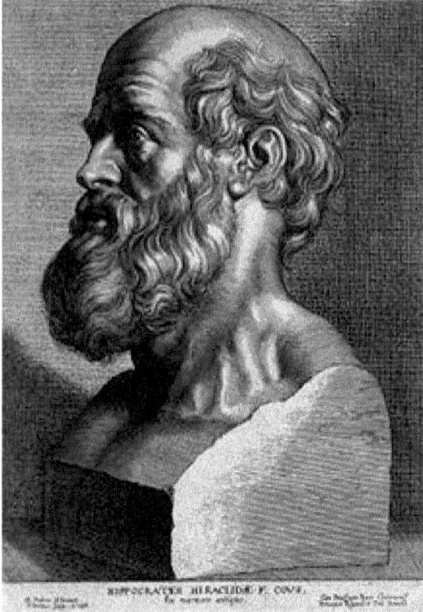

HIPPO'CRATES, the second of that name, and in some respects the most celebrated physician of ancient or modern times ; for not only have his writings (or rather those which bear his name) been always held in the highest esteem, but his personal history (so far as it is known), and the literary criticism relating to his works, furnish so much matter for the consideration both of the scholar, the philologist, the philosopher, and the man of letters, that there are few authors of antiquity about whom so much has been written. Probably the readers of this work will care more for the literary than for the medical questions connected with Hippocrates ; and accordingly (as it is quite impossible to discuss the whole subject fully in these pages) the strictly scientific portion of this article occupies less space than the critical ; and this arrangement in this place the writer is inclined to adopt the more readily, because, while there are many works which contain a good account of the scientific merits of the Hippocratic writings, he is not aware of one where the many literary problems arising from them have been at once fully discussed and satisfactorily determined. This task he is far from thinking that he has himself accomplished, but it is right to give this reason for treating the scientific part of the subject much less fully than he would have done had he been writing for a professed medical work.

A parallel has more than once been drawn be- tween " the Father of Medicine " and " the Father of Poetry ; " and, indeed, the resemblances between the two, both in their personal and literary historj', are so evident, that they could hardly fail to strike any one who was even moderately familiar with classical and medical literature. With respect to their personal history, the greatest uncertainty exists, and our real knowledge is next to nothing ; although in the case of both personages, we have professed lives written by ancient authors, which, however, only tend to show still more plainly the ignorance that prevails on the

subject. Accordingly, as might be expected, fable has been busy in supplying the deficiencies of history, and was for a time fully believed ; till
•sX length a re-action fol- lowed, and an unreasoning credulity was
succeeded by an equally unreasonable scepticism, which reached its
climax when it was boldly asserted that neither Homer nor Hippocrates
had ever ex- istfid. (See Ilouclart, Etudes sur IJifypocrate^ p. 6G0.) The
few facts respecting him that may be considered as tolerably well
ascertained may be told in few words. His father was Ileracleides, who
was also a physician, and belonged to the family of the Asclepiadae.
According to Soraniis (Vita Hippocr.^ in Ilippocr. Opera, vol. iii.), he
was the nineteenth in descent from Aesculapius, but John Tzetzes, who
gives the genealogy of the family, makes him the seventeenth. His
niotlier's name was Phaenarete, who was said to be descended from
Hercules. Soranus, on tlie autho- rity of an old writer who had
composed a life of Hippocrates, states that he was born in the island of
Cos, in the first year of the eightieth Olympiad, that is. B. c. 460 ; and
this date is generally followed, for want of any more satisfactory
inform- ation on the subject, though it agrees so ill with some of the
anecdotes respecting him, that some persons suppose hira to have been
born about thirty years sooner. The exact day of his birth was known
and celebrated in Cos with sacrifices on the '26th. day of the month
Agrianus,but it is unknown to what date in any other calendar this
month cor- responds. He was instructed in medical science by his
father and by Herodicus, and is also said to have been a pupil of
Gorgias of Leontini. He wrote, taught, and practised his profession at
home ; travelled in different parts of the continent of Greece ; and died
at Larissa in Thessaly. His age at the time of his death is uncertain, as it
is stated by different ancient authors to have been eighty-five years,
ninety, one hundred and four, fend one hundred and nine. Mr. Clinton
places his death B. c. 357, at the age of one hundred and four. He had
two sons, Thessalus and Dracon, and a son-in-law, Polybus, all of
whom followed the same profession, and who are supposed to have
been the authors of some of the works in the Hippocratic Collection.
Such are the few and scanty facts that can be in some degree depended
on respecting the personal history of this cele- brated man ; but though
we have not the means of writing an authentic detailed biography, we
possess in these few facts, and in the hints and allusions con- tained in
various ancient authors, sufficient data to enable us to appreciate the
part he played, and the place he held among his contemporaries. We
find that he enjoyed their esteem as a practitioner, writer, and

professor; that he conferred on the ancient and illustrious family to which he belonged more honour than he derived from it ; that he rendered the medical school of Cos, to which he was attached, superior to any which had preceded it or immediately followed it ; and that his works, soon after their publication, were studied and quoted by Plato. (See Littre's Hippocr. vol. i. p. 43 ; and a review of that work (by the writer of this article) in the Brit, and For. Med. Rev. April, 1844, p. 459.)

Upon this slight foundation of historical truth has been built a vast superstructure of fabulous error ; and it is curious to observe how all these tales receive a colouring from the times and coun- tries in which they appear to have been fabricated, whether by his own countrymen before the Chris- tian era, or by the Latin or Arabic writers of the middle ages. One of the stories told of him by his Greek biograpners, which most modern critics are disposed to regard as fabulous, relates to his being sent for, together with Euryphon [EuRV- phon], by Perdiccas II., king of Macedonia, and discovering, by certain external symptoms, that his sickness was occasioned by his having fallen in love with his father's concubine. Probably the strongest reason against the truth of this story is the fact that the time of the supposed cure is quite irreconcileable with the commonly received date of the birth of Hippocrates ; though M. Litire, the latest and best editor of Hippocrates, while he rejects the story as spurious, finds no difficulty in the dates (vol. i. p. 38). Soranus, who tells tlie anecdote, says that the occurrence took place after the death of Alexander I., the father of Perdiccas; and we may rcasonabl} *presume that one or two* years would be the longest interval that would elapse. The date of the death of Alexander is not exactly known, and depends upon the length of the reign of his son Perdiccas, who died b. c. 414. The longest period assigned to his reign is forty- one years, the shortest is twenty-three. This latter date would place his accession to the throne on his father's death, at B. c. 437, at which time Hippo- crates would be only twenty-three years old, almost too young an age for him to have acquired so great celebrity as to be specially sent for to attend a foreign prince. However, the date of B. c. 437 is the less probable because it would not only extend the reign of his father Alexander to more than sixty years, but would also suppose him to have lived seventy years after a period at which he was already grown up to manhood. For these reasons Mr. Clinton {F. Hell. ii. 222) agrees with Dodwell in supposing the longer periods assigned to his reign to be nearer the truth ; and assumes the ac- cession of Perdiccas to have fallen within B. c. 454, at which time Hippocrates was only six years old. This celebrated story has been told, with more or less variation, of Erasistratus and Avicenna, besides being interwoven in the romance of Heliodorus (Aet/dop. iv, 7. p. 171), and the love-letters of Aristaenetus (Epist. i. 13). Galen also says that a similar circumstance happened to himself. (De Praenot. ad Epig. c. 6. vol. xiv. p. 630.) The story as applied to Avicenna seems to be most probably apocryphal (see Biogr. Diet, of the Usef. Knowl. Soc. vol. iv. p. 301) ; and with respect to the two other claimants, Hippocrates and Erasistratus, if it be true of either, the pre- ponderance of historical testimony is decidedly in favour of the latter. [Erasistratus.] Another old Greek fable relates to his being appointed librarian at Cos, and burning the books there (or, according to another version of the story, at Cnidos,) in order to conceal the use he had made of them in his own writings. This story is also told, with but little variation, of Avicenna, and is repeated of Hippocrates, with some characteristic embellish- ments, in the European Legends of the Middle Ages. [Andrkas.]

The other fables concerning Hippocrates are to be traced to the collection of Letters, &c. which go under his name, but which are universally rejected as spurious. The most celebrated of these relates to his supposed conduct during the plague of Athens, which he is said to have stopped by burn- ing fires throughout the city, by suspending chap- lets of flowers, and by the use of an antidote, the composition of which is preserved by Joannes Ac- tuarius {De Meth. Med. v. 6. p. 264, ed. H. Steph.) Connected with this, is the pretended letter from Artaxerxes Longimanus, king of Persia, to Hippocrates, inviting him by great offers to come to his assistance during a time of pestilence, and the re- fusal of Hippocrates, on the ground of his being the enemy of his country.

Another story, perhaps equally familiar to the readers of Burton's "Anatomy of Melancholy," contains the history of the supposed madness of Democritus, and his interview with Hippocrates, who had been sunnnoned by his countrymen to come to his relief.

If we turn to the Arabic writers, we find " Bokrdt " represented as living at Hems, and studying in a garden near Damascus, the situation of which was still pointed out in the time of Abu-1- faraj in the thirteenth century. (Abu-1-faraj, Hist. Dynast, p. 56; Anon. Arab. Philosoph. Bibl. apud Casiri, Bihlioth. A rahico-Hisp. Escur. vol. i. p. 235.) They also tell a story of his pupils taking his por- trait to a celebrated physiognomist named Phile- mon., in order to try his skill ; and that upon his saying that it was the portrait of a lascivious old man (which they strenuously denied), Hippocrates said that he was right, for that he was so by nature, but that he had learned to overcome his amorous propensities. The confusion of names that occurs in this last anecdote the writer has never seen explained, though the difficulty admits of an easy and satisfactory solution. It will no doubt have brought to the reader's recollection the similar story told of Socrates by Cicero (Tusc. Disp. iv. 37, De Fata., c. 5), and accordingly he will be quite prepared to hear that the Arabic writers have confounded the word]b^ JL«j Sokrut^ with ^^ Jj Boki-at., and have thus applied to Hippocrates an anecdote that in reality belongs to Socrates. The name of the physiognomist in Cicero is Zopyrus, which cannot have been corrupted into Philemon ; but when we remember that the Arabians have no /*, and are therefore often obliged to express this letter by an F^ it will probably appear not unlikely that either the writers, or their European trans- lators, have confounded Philemon with Polemon. This conjecture is confirmed by the fact that Phile- mon is said by Abu-1-faraj to have written a work on Physiognomy, which is true of Polemon, whose treatise on that subject is still extant, whereas no person of the name of Philemon (as far as the writer is aware) is mentioned as a physiognomist by any Greek author.* The only objection to this conjecture is the anachronism of making Pole- mon a contemporary of Hippocrates or Socrates ; but this difficulty will not appear very great to any one who is familiar with the extreme igno- rance and carelessness displayed by the Arabic writers on all points of Greek history and chro- nology.

It is, however, among the European story- tellers of the middle ages that the name of " Ypo- cras " is most celebrated. In one story he is repre- sented as visiting Rome during the reign of Au- gustus, and restoring to life the emperor's nephew, who was just dead ; for which service Augustus

- There is at this present time among the MSS.

at Leyden a little Arabic treatise on Physiognomy which bears the name of Philemon., and which (as the writer has been informed by a gentleman who has compared the two works) bears a very great resemblance to the Greek treatise by Polemon. {JXQ Catal. Biblioth. Lujdun. p. 461. § 1286.)

erected a statue in his honour as to a divinity. A fair lady resolved to prove that this god was a mere mortal ; and, accordingly, having made an assignation with him, she let down for him a basket from her window. When she had raised him half way, she left him suspended in the air all night, till he was found by the emperor in the morning, and thus became the laughing-stock of the court. Anoiher story makes him professor of medicine in Rome, with a nephew of wondrous talents and medical skill, whom he despatched in his own stead to the king of Hungary, who had sent for him to heal his son. The young leech, by his marvellous skill, having discovered that the prince was not the king's own son, directed him to feed on " contrarius drink, contrarius mete, beves flesch, and drink the broth t," and thereby soon restored him to health. Upon his return home laden with presents, " Ypocras" became so jealous of his fame, that he murdered him, and afterwards " he let all his bokes berne." The vengeance of Heaven overtook him, and he died in dreadful torments, confessing his crime, and vainly calling on his murdered nephew for relief. (See Ellis, Spec, of Early Engl. Metr. Roman, vol. iii. p. 39 ; Weber, Metr. Rom. of the Wi, Uh, and bth Cent.., ^c, vol. iii. p. 41 ; Way, Fabliaux or Talcs of the ih and 'Mh Cent.^ ^c. vol. ii. p. 173 ; Le- grand d'Aussy, Fabliaux ou Contes, Fables et Ro- mans du eme et du ?>eme Siecles, tome i. p. 288 ; Loiseleur Deslongchamps, Essai sur les Fables Ind. ^c, p. 154, and Roman des Sept Sages, p. 26.)

If, from the personal history of Hippocrates, we turn to the collection of writings that go under his name, the parallel with Homer will be still more exact and striking. In both cases we find a number of works, the most ancient, and, in some respects, the most excellent of their kind, which, though they have for centuries borne the same name, are discovered, on the most cursory examination, to belong in reality to several different persons. Hence has arisen a question which has for ages exercised the learning and acuteness of scholars and critics, and which is in both cases still far from being satisfactorily settled. With respect to the writings of the Hippocratic Collection " the first glance," says M. Littre (vol. i. p. 44), *' shows that some are complete in themselves, while others are merely collections of notes, which follow each other without connection, and which are sometimes hardly intelligible. Some are incomplete and fragmentary, others form in the whole Collection particular series, which belong to the same ideas and the same writer. In a word, however little we reflect ou the context of these numerous writings, we are led to conclude that they are not the work of one and the same author. This remark has in all ages struck those persons who have given their atten- tion to the works of Hippocrates ; and even at the time when men commented on them in the Alex- andrian school, they already disputed about their authenticity."

But it is not merely from internal evidence (though this of itself would be sufficiently con- vincing) that we find that the Hippocratic Collec- tion is not the work of Hippocrates alone, for it so happens that in two insUinces we find a passage that has appeared from very early times as forming part of this collection, quoted as belonging to a dilfereut person. Indeed if we had nothing but internal evidence to guide us in our task of ex- amining these writings, in order to decide which really belong to Hippocrates, we should come to but few positive results ; and therefore it is neces- sary to collect all the ancient testimonies that can still be found ; in doing which, it will appear that the Collection, as a whole, can be traced no higher than the period of the Alexandrian school, in the third century b. c. ; but that particular treatises are referred to by the contemporaries of Hippocrates and his immediate successors. {^Brit. and For. Med. Rev. p. 460.)

We find that Hippocrates is mentioned or re- ferred to by no less than ten persons anterior to the foundation of the Alexandrian school, and among them by Aristotle and Plato. At the time of the formation of the great Alexandrian library, the different treatises which bear the name of Hip- pocrates were diligently sought for, and formed into a single collection ; and about this time commences the series of Commentators, which has continued through a period of more than two thousand years to the present day. The first person who is known to have commented on any of the works of the Hippocratic Collection is Herophilus. [Herophi- Lus.] The most ancient commentary still in ex- istence is that on the treatise " De Articulis," by ApoUonius Citiensis. [Apollonius Citiensis.] By far the most voluminous, and at the same time by far the most valuable commentaries that remain, are those of Galen, who wrote several works in illustration of the writings of Hippocrates, besides those which we now possess. His Commentaries, which are still extant, are those on the " De Na- tura Hominis," " De Salubri Victus Ratione," " De Ratione Victus in Morbis Acutis," " Praenotiones," " Praedictiones I.," " Aphorismi," " De Morbis Vulgaribus I. II. III. VI," " De Fracturis," "De Articulis," " De OfRcina Medici," and " De Hu- moribus," with a glossary of difficult and obsolete words, and fragments on the " De Aere, Aquis, et Locis," and " De Alimento." The other ancient commentaries that remain are those of Palladius, Joannes Alexandrinus, Stephanus Atheniensis, Meletius, Theophilus Protospatharius, and Damas- cius ; besides a spurious work attributed to Ori- basius, a glossary of obsolete and difficult words by I'lrotianus, and some Arabic Commentaries that have never been published. {^Brit. and For. Med. Rev. p. 461.)

His writings were held in the highest esteem by the ancient Greek and Latin physicians, and most of them were translated into Arabic. (See Wen- rich, De Auct. Grace. Vers, et Comment. Syr. Arab., &c.) In the middle ages, however, they were not so much studied as those of some other authors, whose works are of a more practical cha- racter, and better fitted for being made a class-book and manual of instruction. In more modern times, on the contrary, the works of the Hippocratic Col- lection have been valued more according to their real worth, while many of the most popular medical writers of the middle ages have fallen into complete neglect. The number of works written in illustra- tion or explanation of the Collection is very great, as is also that of the editions of the whole or any part ol the treatises composing it. Of these only a very few can be here mentioned : a fuller account may be found in Fabric. Bibl. Grace. ; Haller, Bibl. Medic. Pract.; the first vol. of Kiihn's edi- tion of Hippocrates; Choulanfs Ilandb. der Bu- clierTcunde fur die Aellere Medicin ; Littre's Hip- pocrates ; and other professed bibliographical works. 'J'he works of Hippocrates first appeared in a Latin translation by Fabius Calvus, Rom. 1525, fol. The first Greek edition is the Aldine, Venet. 1526, fol., which was printed from MSS. with hardly any correction of the transcriber's errors. The first edition that had any pretensions to be called a critical edition was that by Hieron. Mercurialis, Venet. 1588, fol., Gr. and Lat. ; but this was much surpassed by that of Anut. Foesius, Francof. 1595, fol., Gr. and Lat., which continues to the present day to be the best complete edition. Van- der Linden's edition (Lugd. Bat. 1 665, 8vo. 2 vols. Gr. and Lat.) is neat and commodious for refer- ence from his having divided the text into short paragraphs. Chartier's edition of the works of Galen and Hippocrates has been noticed under Galen; as has also Kiihn's, of which it may be said that its only advantages are its convenient size, the reprint of Ackermann's Histor. Liter. Hippocr. (from Harless's ed. of Fabr. Bibl. Gr.) in the first vol., and the noticing on each page the cor- responding pagination of the editions of Foes, Chartier, and Vander Linden. By far the best edition in every respect is one which is now in the course of publication at Paris, under the super- intendence of E. Littre, of which the first vol. ap- peared in 1839, and the fourth in 1844. It contains a new text, founded upon a collation of the MSS. in the Royal Library at Paris ; a French translation ; an interesting and learned general In- troduction, and a copious argument prefixed to each treatise ; and numerous scientific and philological notes. It is a work quite indispensable to every physician, critic, and philologist, who wishes to study in detail the works of the Hippocratic Col- lection, and it has already done much more to- wards settling the text than any edition that has preceded it ; but at the same time it must not be concealed that the editor does not seem to have always made the best use of the materials that he has had at his command, and that the classical reader cannot help now and then noticing a mani- fest want of critical (and even at times of gram- matical) scholarship.

The Hippocratic Collection consists of more than sixty works ; and the classification of these, and assigning each (as far as possible) to its proper author, constitutes by far the most diffi- cult question connected with the ancient medical writers. Various have been the classifications proposed both in ancient and modem times, and various the rules by which their authors were guided ; some contenting themselves with following implicitly the opinions of Galen and Erotianus, others arguing chiefly from peculiarities of style, while a tliird class distinguished the books accord- ing to the medical and philosophical doctrines contained in them. An account of each of these classifications cannot be given here, much less can the objections that may be brought against each be pointed out : upon the whole, the writer is inclined to think M. Littre's superior to any that has pre- ceded it ; but by no means so imexceptionable as to do away with the necessity of a new one. The following classification, though far enough from supplying the desideratum, difi'ers in several in- stances from any former one : it is impossible here for the writer to give more than the results of his investigation, referring for the data on which hia opinion in each particular case is founded to the works of Gniner, Ackermann, and Littre, of which he has, of course, made free use.* Perhaps a tabular or genealogical view of the different divisions and subdivisions of the Collection will be the best cal- culated to put the reader at once in possession of the whole bearings of the subject.

The Hippocratic Collection consists of Works certainltf ■written by Hip- pocrates. (Class Works certainly not written by Hippocrates. Works perhaps written by Hip- pocrates. (Class ll.) Works earliei than Hippo- crates. (Class III.) Works later than Hippo- crates. Works about contemporary with Hippo- crates. I >Vorks authentic, but not genuine, i. e. not wilful forgeries. Works neither genuine nor authentic, i.e. wilful forge- ries. (Class VIII.) I I Works whose Works whose author is author is conjectured. unknown. (Class IV.) (Class V.) Works by va- rious authors. (Class VII.) Works by the same author. (Class VI.)

Class I., containing UpoyuaxTTiKdv, Praenotiones or Prognosticon (vol. i. p. 88, ed. Kiihn) ; 'A^o- pia-fiol, Aphorismi (vol. iii. p. 706) ; 'EiridTjixicou Bi§ia A, r, De Morbis Popularilms (or Epidemi- orum lib. i. and iii. (vol. i. pp. 382, 467) ; Hept AjaiTTjs 'O|6ojj', De Ratione Victus in Morbis Acutis, or De Diaeta Acutorum (vol. ii. p. 25); Tlepi *Aepiou^ 'TSdruv^ Tottwv, De Acre, Aquisy et Locis (vol. i. p, 523) ; Uepl twu kv KecpoKfj Tpu- ixdruu, De Capitis Vulneribus (vol. iii. p. 346).

Class II., containing Ilepl "Apxaf-ns 'iTjTpj/crjy, De Prisca Medidna (vol. i. p. 22) ; Hep! "Apdpwv, De Articidis (vol. iii. p. 135); Uepl ^KyixSv^ De Fradis (vol. iii. p. 64); MoxA.tKos, MochUms or Vectiarius (vol. iii. p. 270) ; "OpKos, Jicsjurandum (vol. i. p. 1) ; ^o/xos. Lex (vol. i. p. 3); llepl 'E/c(Sj', De Ulceribus (vol. iii. p. 307) ; Tl^pX ^vpiyywv^ De Fistulis (vol. iii. p. 329); Uepl AtfjLo^pot^cov^ De Haemorrhoidibus (o. iii. p. 340); KaT* 'iTjrpetoj', De Officina Medici (vol. iii. p. 48) ; TlepX 'Iprjs Uovaov^ De Morbo Sacra (vol. i. p. 587).

Class III., containing Tlpo^f)7}riK6v A, Pror- rlietica^ or Praedidiones i. (vol. i. p. 157) ; KcoaKot npoyvdaeis, Coacae Praenotiones (vol. i. p. 234).

Class IV., containing Uspl ^vcrios 'Avdpciirov, De Natura Hominis (vol. i. p. 348) ; riepl Aiairrts "Tyieivrjs, De Salubri Victus Ratione {?) (vol. i. p. 616); riepl TouaiK^i-n^ ^uaios, De Natura Mu- liebri(?) (vol. ii. p. 529) ; Uepl Nomwv B, T, De Morbis, ii. iii(?) (volii. p.212); Uepl 'EmKv^<rios, De Super/oetatione{?) (vol. i. p. 460).

Class v., containing Uepl Ouawi', De Phtibus (vol. i. p. 569) ; Uepl TSituv twv kut "AvOpwrrov^ De Locis in Homine (vol. ii. p. 101) ; Ilepl Texi'Tjy, De Arte{?) (vol. i. p. 5) ; Uepl AiatTijs, De Diaeta, or De Victus Ratione (vol. i. p. 625) ; Uepl 'Ei/u-

- Some of the readers of this work may perhaps

be interested to hear that a strictly ;)A«7o/or/2ca/ clas- sification of the works of the Hippocratic Collection is still a desideratum ; and that, as this is in fact almost the only question connected with the subject which has not by this time been thoroughly ex- amined, any scholar who will undertake the work will be doing good service to the cause of ancient medical literature.

■npltav, De Insomniis (vol. ii. p. 1); Uepl UaOwv, De Affectionibus (vol. ii. p. 380) ; Uepl tcov evros UadoSu, De Internis Affectionilms (vol. ii. p. 427) ; Uepl Novaav A, De Morbis i. (vol. ii. p. 1 65) ; Uepl 'EirTajj-riuov, De Septimestri Partu (vol. i. p. 444) ; Uepl 'OKTafxrivov, De Octimestri Partu (vol. i. p. 455) ; ^EiTi8'r]ixi(av Bi§la B, A, Z, Epidemiorum, or De Morbis Popularibtis, ii. iv. vi. (vol. iii. pp. 428, 511, 583) ; Uepl Xv/jlu/v, De Ilumoribus (vol. i. p. 120) ; Uepl 'Typwv Xpijaios, De Usu Liqui- dorum (vol. ii. p. 153).

Class VI., containing Uepl Vovrs, De Genitura (vol. i. p. 371) ; Uepl ^va-ios UaiSiov, De Natura Pueri (vol. i. p. 382) ; Ilepl 'No^awv A, De Morbis iv. (vol. ii. p. 324) ; Uepl TuvaiKeim', De Mu- lierum Morbis (vol. ii. p. 606) ; Utpl Uap6ei>iw}/, De Virginum Morbis (vol. ii. p. 526) ; Uepl 'A(p6- puiv, De Sterilibus (vol. iii. p. 1).

Class VII., containing 'EttjStJjUiwi' BigAta E, H, Epidemiorum, or De Morbis Popularibus v. vii. fvol. iii. pp. 545, 631) ; UeX KapStTjy, De Corde (vol. i. p. 485) ; Ilept Tpo<pT/s, De Alimento (vol. ii. p. 17) ; Ilept ^dpKoou, De Carnibus (vol. i. p. 424); Uepl 'ESSofjidSuv, De Septimanis, a work which no longer exists in Greek, but of which M. Littr6 has found a Latin translation ; Upop^rjTiKou B, Prorrhetica (or

Praedidiones) ii. (vol. i. p. 185) ; Uepl 'Oa-Tewu ^vcrios, De Natura Ossium, a work composed entirely of extracts from other treatises of the Hippocratic Collection, and from other an- cient authors, and which therefore M. Littre is going to suppress entirely (vol. i. p. 502) ; Uepl 'ASevwu, De Glandtdis (vol. i. p. 491); Uepl 'iTjTpov, De Medico (vol. i. p. 56) ; Uepl Ev- o'XVfJ-oavvTjs, De Decenti Habitu (vol. i. p. 66) ; UapayyeXiai, Praeceptiones (vol. i. p. 77) ; Uepl 'AvaTopLris, De Anatomia (or De Resedione Cor- porum) (vol. iii. p. 379) ; Uepl 'OSourocpvi'-ns, De Dmtitione (vol. i. p. 482) ; Uepl ^Ey Kararojxris 'E/i- Spvov, De Resedione Foetus (vol. iii. p. 376) ; Uepl "Oxl/ios, De Visu (vol. iii. p. 42) ; Uepl Kpialcau, De Crisibus (or De Judicationibus) (vol. i. p. 136) ; Uepl Kpiaifxwu, De Diebus Criticis (or De Diebus Judicatortis) (vol. i. p. 149) ; Uepl ^apixoLKoav, De Medicamentis Purgativis (vol. iii. p. 855 j.

Class VIII., containing 'EtnaroKal, Epistolae (vol. iii. p. 769) ; UpecrSevrinos ©eaaaXou, Tlies- sali Legati Oratio (vol. iii. p. 831); 'Etv iSoifxios, Oratio ad Aram (vol. iii. p. 830) ; Aoyjxa 'AOrj- vaicov, Atlieniensium Senatus Consultum (vol. iii. p. 829).

Each of these classes requires a few words of explanation. The first class will probably be con- sidered by many persons to be rather small ; but it seemed safer and better to include in it only those works of whose genuineness there has never been any doubt. To this there is perhaps one ex- ception, and that relating to the very work whose genuineness one would perhaps least expect to find called in question, as it is certainly that by which Hippocrates is most popularly known. Some doubts have arisen in the minds of several eminent critics as to the origin of the Aphorisms, and indeed the discussion of the genuineness of this work may be said to be an epitome of the questions relating to the whole Hippocratic Collection. We find here a very celebrated work, which has from early times borne the name of Hippocrates, but of which some parts have always been condemned as spurious. Upon examining tliose portions that are considered to be genuine, we observe that the greater part of the first three sections agrees almost word for word with passages to be found in his acknowledged works ; while in the remaining sections we find sentences fciken apparently from spurious or doubt- ful treatises ; thus adding greatly to our difficulties, inasmuch as they sometimes contain doctrines and theories opposed to those which we find in the works acknowledged to be genuine. And these facts are (in the opinion of the critics alluded to) to be accounted for in one of two ways : either Hippocrates himself in his old age (for the Apho- risms have always been attributed to this period of his life) put together certain extracts from his own works, to which were afterwards added other sen- tences taken from later authors ; or else the col- lection was not formed by Hippocrates himself, but by some person or persons after his death, who made aphoristical extracts from his works, and from those of other writers of a later date, and the whole was then attributed to Hippocrates, because he was the author of the sentences that were most valuable, and came first in order. This account of the formation of the Aphorisms appears extremely plausible, nor does it seem to be any decisive ob- jection to say, that we find among them sentences which are not to be met with elsewhere ; for, when we recollect how many works of the old medical writers, and perhaps of Hippocrates himself, are lost, it is easy to conceive that these sentences may have been extracted from some treatise that is no longer in existence. It must however be con- fessed that this conjecture, however plausible and probable, requires further proof and examination before it can be received as true.

The second class is one of the most unsatisfac- tory in the writers own opinion, and affords at the same time a curious instance of the impossibility of satisfying even those few persons in Europe whose opinion on such a matter is really worth asking ; fi)r, upon submitting the classification to two friends, one of whom is decidedly the most learned phy- sician in Great Britain, and the other one of the best medical critics on the continent, he was ad- vised by the one to call this class "Works probably written by Hippocrates," and by the other to trans- fer them (with one exception) to the class of

- ' Works certainly not written by Hippocrates."

The amount of probability in favour of the genuine- ness of all these works is certainly by no means equal ; e. g. the two little pieces called the " Oath," and thS " Law," though commonly considered to be the work of the same author, and to be in- timately connected with each other, seem rather to belong to different periods, the former having all the simplicity, honesty, and religious feeling of an- tiquity, the latter somewhat of the affectation and declamatory grandiloquence of a sophist. How- ever, as all of these books have been considered to be genuine by some critics of more or less note, it seemed better to defer to their authority at least 80 far as to allow that they might perhaps have been written by Hippocrates himself.

The two works which constitute the third class, and which are probably the oldest medical writings that exist, have been supposed with some proba- bility to consist, at least in part, of the inscriptions on the votive tablets placed in the temple of Aescu- lapius by those who had recovered their health, which certJiinly constituted one of the sources from which the medical knowledge of Hippocrates was derived.

In the fourth class are placed those works which were certainly not written by Hippocrates himself, which were probably either contemporary or but little posterior to him, and whose authors have been, with more or less degree of certainty, dis- covered. The works De Natura Hoini/ns, and I)e Salubri Victus Ratmie^ are supposed by M. Littre to have been written by the same author, because it is said by Galen that in many old editions these two treatises formed but one ; and this author he concludes to have been Polybus, the son-in-law of Hippocrates (vol. i. pp. 46, 316, &c.), because a passage is quoted by Aristotle {Hist. Aiiiin. .iii ?>), and attributed to Polybus, which is found word for word in the work De Natura Iluminis (vol. i. p. 364). For somewhat similar reasons, Euryphon has been supposed to be the author of the second and third books De Morbis, and the work De Natura Muliebri [Euryphon] ; and also (though with much less show of reason) a certain Leo- phanes, or Cleophanes (of whom nothing whatever is known), to have written the treatise De Sujxrr- foetatione (Littr^, vol. i p. 380).

In the fifth class there is one treatise {De Di- aeta) in which an astronomical, coincidence with the calendar of Eudoxus has been pointed to the writer by a friend, which (as far as he is aware) has never been noticed by any commentator on Hippocrates, and which seems in some degree to fix the date of the work in question. If the ca- lendar of Eudoxus, as preserved in the Ajyparentiae of Ptolemy and the calendar of Geminus (see Petav. Uranol. pp. 64, 71), be compared with part of the third book De Diaeta (vol. i. pp. 7 1 1 —7 1 5), it will be found that the periods correspond so exactly, that (there being no other solar calendar of antiquity in which these intervals coincide so closely,and all through,but that of Eudoxus), it seems a reasonable inference that the writer of the work De Diaeta took them from the calendar in question. If this be granted, it will follow that the author must have written this work after the year B. c. 381, which is the date of the calendar of Eu- doxus ; and, as Hippocrates must have been at least eighty years old at that time, this conclusion will agree quite well with the general opinion of ancient and modern critics, that the treatise in question was probably written by one of his im- mediate followers.

The sixth class agrees with the sixth class of M. Littr^, who, with great appearance of proba- bility, supposes it to form a connected series of works written by the same author, whose name is quite unknown, and of whose date it can only be determined from internal evidence that he must have lived later than Hippocrates, and before the time of Aristotle.

The works contained in this and the seventh class have for many centuries formed part of the Hippocratic Collection without having any right to such an honour, and therefore are not genuine ; but, as it does not appear that their authors were guilty of assuming the name of Hippocrates, or that they have represented the state of medical science as in any respect different from what it really was in the times in which they wrote, there is no reason for denying their authenticity. And in this respect they are to be regarded with a very different eye from the pieces which form the last class, which are neither genuine nor authentic, but mere forgeries ; which display indeed here and there some ingenuity and skill, but which are still sufficiently full of difficulties and inconsistencies to betray at once their origin.

So much space has been taken up with the pre- liminary, but most indispensable step of determin- ing which are the genuine works of Hippocrates, and which are spurious, that a very slight sketch of his opinions is all that can be now attempted, and for a fuller account the reader must be referred to the works of Le Clerc, Haller, Sprengel, &c., or to some of those which relate especially to Hippo- crates, He divides the causes of disease into two principal classes ; the one comprehending the in- fluence of seasons, climates, water, situation, &c., and the other consisting of more personal and pri- vate causes, such as result from the particular kind and amount of food and exercise in which each separate individual indulges himself. The modifi- cations of the atmosphere dependent on different seasons and climates is a subject which was suc- cessfully treated by Hippocrates, and which is still far from exhausted by all the researches of modern science. He considered that while heat and cold, moisture and dryness, succeeded one another throughout the year, the human body underwent certain analogous changes, which influenced the diseases of the period ; and on this basis was founded the doctrine of pathological constitutions, corresponding to particular conditions of the at- mosphere, so that, whenever the year or the season exhibited a special character in which such or such a temperature prevailed, those persons who were exposed to its influence were affected by a series of disorders, all bearing the same stamp. (How plainly the same idea runs through the Observaii- ones Medicae of Sydenham, our *English Hippo-crates* " need not be pointed out to those who are at all familiar with his works.) Tlie belief in the influence which different climates exercise on the human frame follows naturally from the theory just mentioned ; for, in fact, a climate may be con- sidered as nothing more than a permanent season, whose effects may be expected to be more power- ful, inasmuch as the cause is ever at work upon mankind. Accordingly, Hippocrates attributes to climate both the conformation of the body and the disposition of the mind — indeed, almost every thing ; and if the Greeks were found to be hardy freemen, and the Asiatics effeminate slaves, he accounts for the difference of their characters by that of the climates in which they lived. With respect to the second class of causes producing disease, he attributed all sorts of disorders to a vicious system of diet, which, whether excessive or defective, he considered to be equally injurious ; and in the same way' he supposed that, when bo- dily exercise was either too much indulged in or entirely neglected, the health was equally likely to suffer, thougli by different forms of disease. Into all the minutiae of the " Humoral Pathology " (as it was called), which kept its ground in FJurope as the prevailing doctrine of all the medical sects for more than twenty centuries, it would be out of place to enter here. It will be sufficient to remind the reader that the four fluids or humours of the body (blood, phlegm, yellow bile, and black bile) were supposed to be the primary seat of disease ; that health was the result of the due combination (or crash) of these, and that, when this crasis was disturbed, disease was the consequence ; that, iu the course of a disorder that was proceeding fa- vourably, these humours underwent a certain change in quality (or coction), which was the sign of returning health, as preparing the way for the expulsion of the morbid matter, or crisis; and that these crises had a tendency to occur at certain stated periods, which were hence called " critical days." {Brit, and For. Med. Rev.)

The medical practice of Hippocrates was cautious and feeble, so much so, that he was in after times reproached with letting his patients die, by doing nothing to keep them alive. It consisted chiefly in watching tiie operations of nature, and pro- moting the critical evacuations mentioned above ; so that attention to diet and regimen was the principal and often the only remedy that he em- ployed. Several hundred substances have been enumerated which are used medicinally in different parts of the Hippocratic Collection ; of these, by far the greater portion belong to the vegetable kingdom, as it would be in vain to look for any traces of chemistry in these early writings. In surgery, he is the author of the frequently quoted maxim, that " what cannot be cured by medicines is cured by the knife ; and what cannot be cured by the knife is cured by fire." The anatomical knowledge displayed in different parts of the Hip- pocratic Collection is scanty and contradictory, so much so, that the discrepancies on this subject constitute an important criterion in deciding the genuineness of the different treatises.

With regard to the personal character of Hip- pocrates, though he says little or nothing expressly about himself, yet it is impossible to avoid drawing certain conclusions from the characteristic passages scattered through the pages of his writings. He was evidently a person who not only had had great experience, but who also knew how to turn it to the best account ; and the number of moral reflections and apophthegms that we meet with in his writings, some of which (as, for example, " Life is short, and Art is long ") have acquired a sort of proverbial notoriety, show him to have been a profound thinker. He appears to have felt the moral obligations and responsibilities of his profession, and often tries to impress upon his readers the duties of care and attention, and kind- ness towards the sick, saying that a physician's first and chief consideration ought to be the re- storing his patient to health. The style of the Hippocratic writings, which are in the Ionic dialect, is so concise as to be sometimes extremely ohscure ; though this charge, which is as old as the time of Galen, is often brought too indiscriminately against the whole collection, whereas it applies, in fact especially only to certain treatises, which seem to be merely a collection of notes, such as De IJu- moribiis, De Alimeido^ De Ojjlcina Medici, &c. In those writings, which are universally allowed to be genuine, we do not find this excessive brevity, though even these are in general by no means easy. {Brit, and For. Med. Rev.)

Of the great number of books published on the subject of the Hippocratic Collection, only a very few of the most modern and most useful can be here enumerated ; a fuller list may be found in Choulant's Handb. der li'ucherkunde fur die Aeltere Medicin, or his Biblioth. Medico- 1 Hi- tor. ; or in Ackermann's Historia Literaria Ilijypo- crutis. Fiiesii Oeco7iomia Ilippocrads is a very copious and learned lexicon, published in fol. Francof. 1588, and Gene v. I(i62. Sprengel'B Apologie des Hippocr. und seiner Grundsatze (Leipz. 1789, 1792, 2 vols. 8vo.), contains, among other matter, a Gennan translation of some of tlie genuine treatises, with a valuable commentary. The treatise by Ermerins, De Hippocr. Doctrina a Prognostice oriunda (Lugd. Bat. 1832, 4to,), de- serves to be carefully studied ; as also does Link's dissertation, Ueher die Theorien in den Hippocra- tisclien Schriften^ nebst Bemerkungen uber die Echt- I/eit dieser ScJinflen^ in the * *Abhandlungen der* Berlin. Akadem.*' 1814, 1815. Gruner's Censura Lil)rorum Hippocraieorum qua veri a fulsis^ intcgri a supj)ositis segreganiur, Vratislav. 1772, 8vo., con- tains a useful account of the amount of evidence in favour of each treatise of the collection, though his conclusions are not always to be depended on. See al«o Houdart, Etudes Histor. et Crit. sur la Vie et kc Doctrine d' Hippocr. Paris, 183G, 8vo.; Petersen, Hippocr. Nomine quae circuiiiferuntur Scripta ad Temporis Raiiones dispos. Hamburg, 1839, 4to. ; Meixner, Neue Prnfung der Eehtlieit und Reiliefolge S'dmmtlicher Schriften Hippocr.^ Miinchen, 1836, 1837, 8vo. [W. A. G.]

www.ingramcontent.com/pod-product-compliance
Lightning Source LLC
Chambersburg PA
CBHW071532210326
41597CB00018B/2978